REDEEMED

An Overcomer's Journey to
Becoming a World Champion

Daniel Stephens

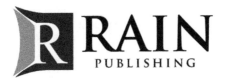

Somerset, NJ

Daniel Stephens/Rain Publishing
www.rainpublishing.com

Edited by: Rachel Renee/Rain Publishing

Redeemed – An Overcomer's Journey to Becoming a World Champion/ Daniel Stephens. -- 1st ed.
ISBN 978-1-7328709-3-2

Library of Congress Control Number: 2019913141

Book Dedicated to my Beloved Grandmother

Lillian Ruby Stephens

REST IN PEACE

&

My Daughter

Isabella Rose Stephens

ACKNOWLEDGMENTS

Special thanks to all my Family, Friends, and Supporters who supported me throughout my career.

<u>WIFE</u>
Megan Elmore Stephens

<u>PARENTS</u>
Alan Stephens
Cyndi Stephens

<u>IN-LAWS</u>
Joe Elmore
Pat Elmore

<u>SIBLINGS</u>
Josh Stephens
Kathryn Stephens
Lauren Elmore Pecci

<u>MENTOR/COACH</u>
BJ Little

SUPPORTERS

Marcel Anderson

Kim Henson

CT Fletcher

Samer Hosn

Dianna Lowry

Josh Miller

Jamie Miller

Megan Hoffman

Jamarcus Gaston

Kit Hemenway Clark

Vicki Graham

OTHERS

Your Carolina

Scene on 7

Anytime Fitness

Spartanburg Athletic

To those not listed, I am still grateful for everyone who supported me through my career and life challenges. It could not have been done without any of your love and gratitude.

"You can't connect the dots looking forward, you can only connect them looking backwards. So you have to trust that the dots will somehow connect in your future.

You have to trust in something: Your gut, destiny, Life, karma, whatever. Because believing that the dots will connect down the road will give you the confidence to follow your heart, even when it leads you off the well-worn path. And that will make all the difference. Your time is limited; so don't waste it living someone else's life. Don't be trapped by dogma — which is living with the results of other people's thinking. Don't let the noise of others' opinions drown out your own inner voice. You've got to find what you love. And that is as true for work as it is for your lovers. Your work is going to fill a large part of your life and the only way to be truly satisfied is to do what you believe is great work. And the only way to do great work is to love what you do. If you haven't found it yet, keep looking, and don't settle. Have the courage to follow your heart and intuition. They somehow already know what you truly want to become"

- Steve Jobs

"The real challenge is growth; mentally, emotionally, spiritually, comes from when you get knocked down. It takes courage to act. Part of being hungry, when you have been defeated, it takes courage to start over again."

-Les Brown

CONTENTS

Young and Relentless

Gentlemen, we are going to relentlessly chase perfection, knowing full well we will not catch it, because nothing is perfect. But we are going to relentlessly chase it, because in the process we will catch excellence. I am not remotely interested in just being good.

~Vince Lombardi

Growing up, I remember being such a perfectionist at everything I did, whether it be a sport I played or just writing my name correctly. My dad got me and my brother involved in baseball and karate at a young age and the one thing he always taught me was to never give up. If I showed one sign of quitting, he would pull me to the side and give me a lecture of a lifetime. He always wanted to see me do my best and wanted me to give my best. Sometimes I would be so nervous that if I screwed up he would be very disappointed in me. That was never the case; if I gave everything I had into whatever I did, he was proud. But he also knew when I was just being plain lazy and that is when he would hammer down on me. I always wanted to please my parents and make them proud.

I never really got the concept of doing what's best for me until I hit high school. The perfectionist in me turned me into a relentless track runner. My parents tried for a couple years to get me to run track because during field days at school, I would always outrun everyone. I had the speed but didn't have the discipline. My eighth-grade year I decided I would go out for the track team. I was not sure what to expect or where I would even start, but I knew I wanted to do sprints. Coach Urban was the head coach at Dorman High School at the time and he tried me at the 200m and 400m dash.

I was this skinny, 110-pound kid with no clue on how to run a race. I just knew one thing and that was I wanted to be the best. That was not the case my first year. I came in dead last every race and could never build enough speed to get my times down. Coach Urban wasn't even sure if I was going to cut it as a track runner, but I refused to quit, and I was so determined to get better. I do not take losing lightly. Being competitive has always been something I took seriously. After my first year was over, it was one of those things where I had two options: to continue to get better or to quit. I chose to continue.

After my first year on the track, because I was so determined, I spent the off season hitting the weights and more time on the track. I refused to come last in another race. From that point on, each year I continued to grow and eventually become one of the top 400m sprinters in the state. My team mates and friends would always have to tell me to rest because I was always on the track in my free time. I became so obsessed with being the best that I would overtrain. It was all I could think about. It was my life.

Going into my senior year I had many goals to obtain, but the main one was that I wanted to be the State Champ 400m sprinter. At this point in my career I was so determined, so focused that I refused to let anyone get in my way. I was winning races and my time had improved so much that I was certain that I could win the State Championships. I was going to win the State Championships! I made sure I put in the extra time at practice and in the weight room to improve my performance. Little did I know I was really hurting myself.

Because I over-trained so much, I caused an injury to my hamstring halfway through my senior year. It put a big dent in my ability to fun raster because I could never seem to get it to heal. I never actually allowed it to heal because I continued to over-train. I remember one morning, and this has always stuck with me, Coach Urban pulled me into his classroom and told me, "You don't win medals for how hard you practice," meaning I needed to stop pushing myself so hard at practice so that I could put it all out on race day.

I created a monster inside of me that stayed hungry and was so determined to be the best. If you were in my way, I was going to come after you and I was going to beat you. There was no letting up and there was no stopping me. I was a force that no one could stop. I refused to give in and quit. That is what made me into the athlete that I became and that is where this story begins.

NOTES

Creating a Vision

Vision without action is merely a dream. Action without vision just passes the time. Vision with action can change the world.

~Joel A. Baker

One of my biggest goals in life was to go to the Olympics as a track runner. I wanted to be the world's fastest 400m runner. During the 2004 Olympic Games there was one particular track star that stood out to me and his name was Jeremy Wariner. Jeremy, much like World Olympic Champion Michael Johnson, was a big stand out amongst the runners. He was the high favorite and I could see myself being in his shoes. He ended up winning the 2004 Olympics in the 400m dash which gave me hope that someday it could be me.

My senior year of high school was a big year for me. I had my first real girlfriend, I was looking at colleges and even looking for track scholarship opportunities to run for a big school. For anyone that knows me I am a huge South Carolina Gamecock fan and that was my main choice. They sent me letters but so did other schools. I even sent in a request to Clemson. The important thing was which school had the better opportunity for me and offered more scholarship.

I always excelled in the classroom. I made good grades and just like on the track I wanted to be my best with my school work. I worked hard all through high school to make sure I kept my grades up so that I could get into a good college. The one thing that held me back was my SAT scores. I have never been a great test taker, nor could I understand many of the questions being asked. I think I got points for spelling my name right, but my low score prevented me from getting into a big school even though I was an A/B honor student.

Life was really good. I had an amazing girlfriend and I had great friends that I hung out with; I really thought my future was looking great and I intended on keeping it that way. I met Samer Hosn freshman year of high school. We immediately became friends and still are to this day; it was a bromance for sure. He was one who always spoke highly of me and supported me no matter what I did. The same with my girlfriend, she was always supportive and there to pick me up when I had a bad race or even having a bad day and I was so appreciative for what I had.

My girlfriend at the time was younger than me. I believe she was a sophomore, so she was a couple years younger, but I knew that when it came time to go to college it was going to be a tough decision on what we should do with our relationship. I was in love with her and thought that shouldn't stop us from staying together and that we would find a way to make it work. Again, she was very supportive. She had a way of making me do great things and making me feel more alive. So, I knew it would be tough leaving her to go off to school. But we talked about it and decided to make it work.

After visiting a couple of schools, I found out because of my SAT scores there was only one school that was willing to offer a scholarship and help me reach my goals of becoming a great track athlete. That school was Lees-McRae College. This school is located in Banner Elk, NC and it was a beautiful campus. I had a great feeling about it, so I took them up on their offer and signed to be a Bobcats track runner.

Needless to say, because of my leg injury I was unable to hit my benchmark of becoming the state champion, but I felt like I was in such a great place that I could continue to grow as I got to college. I remember having a conversation with my dad about if it was something I really wanted to do. Did I really want to keep running in college? It was actually a great question because I had never really thought about it, but I really did want to continue at a higher level of competition. So, I got everything together and headed to Lees-McRae.

NOTES

Expectation vs. Reality

Reality is merely an illusion, albeit a very persistent one.

~Albert Einstein

I can be honest, I was extremely nervous when I was about to start a new chapter in my life. I wasn't sure what to expect when it came to adjusting to a different atmosphere and different way of living. I was becoming an adult on my own and making my own decisions. I was also sad because I was leaving my family, friends, and girlfriend to pursue a dream although I knew they were back home rooting me on and supporting me. I knew it would take time to adjust but I was excited about the new journey I was embarking on, the opportunity I was given to make my dreams come true.

Being a college athlete is a whole different ball game of competition than high school. The practices, the meets, and the athletes are on a higher level and require a higher intensity of training. It took me a few practices to get used to the level of running I was embarking on. We were running in high elevations where if you aren't used to those conditions, you become worn out very quickly. Once I became more confident and adjusted to the new conditions, I had a different mentality. Nothing was going to stop me from being the best and going after my dreams.

The biggest obstacle I had to take on was my blood sugar. In that stage of my life I had to be on a strict diet in order to maintain a normal blood sugar level. If I didn't I would have episodes that were not fun. I would get dizzy, faint, lose strength, and even shake uncontrollably. My mom, bless her heart, worried about this constantly so she would make me home cooked meals. She was the only one who understood what I needed and so she made sure I had the proper snacks and meals. I had a couple of episodes that I had to get over but for the most part, I was able to maintain my levels.

Once the season started I was doing well for the most part keeping up with the new level of competition. I knew it would take more than over night to become a success at the college level, but that didn't mean I wasn't going to give it my all and go after it. What most people don't understand either is when you are at that level of competition, your strategies change and your mindset changes. Adapting to new levels of competition can affect the level of stress you put on your mind and your body. During one meet, I let stress get the best of me. I was halfway through a race and because my stress levels were so high, it took a lot out of me causing me to pass out. My blood sugar levels had dropped.

This race determined my spot on the team for the regional cross country meet. Because I did not finish the race, the coach simply told me he did not think I would be able to compete for the regional meet, so he put someone else in my spot. Being the relentless person I was, I did not like hearing that. I do not like being told what I will and will not be able to do. That caused me to push myself even harder to earn my spot back on the team for that particular meet. I knew if I was going to prove myself, it was going to have to be on this particular speed day.

The day came where we had speed work and I was determined to take back my spot. I can't remember the exact distance we ran but it was something like 1,000 meters. With each 1,000 meter race I pushed more and more; I wasn't going to be told I am not doing this meet. Each repeat I got faster and more fired up. I was on fire that day. I had the best times and the most consistent times during that workout that the coach put me back in the regional race. He looked at me and told me, "I want you to bring that race to its mother f***ing knees!" And that is exactly what I did!

NOTES

A Vicious Hit

*Life has many ways of testing a person's will,
either by having nothing happen at all or by
having everything happen all at once.*

~Paulo Coelho

Being such a strong and relentless individual in
sports, I never thought anything could bring me
down. I thought I was unstoppable. If I got knocked
down, I got back up and came back even stronger.
But one of my biggest weaknesses was talking out
my thoughts and feelings. I allowed everyone to
walk all over me because I was such a nice person. I
fell in the pushover category. Other than that, I was
such a strong person, or so I thought. After having a
decent start to college athletics and becoming more
confident in being a stronger runner, it was time to
head home for winter break and that is when everything started to take a turn for the worse.

At the time my grandmother, my father's mother,
was living with my parents. My grandmother had
back surgery when I got home for winter break and
so with me being home I was able to keep an eye on

her. On December 20th, my grandmother's birthday, it was just me and her. I would usually check on her from time to time, but on this day, for whatever reason, I stayed in my room all day. I only came out to eat and check the mail. Well that night, I was sitting in my room playing video games, and my dad came rushing into my room asking me if I knew what happened to my grandmother. Turns out, my grandmother had a stroke.

My mind started racing. I had never dealt with anything like this, and I was scared. They rushed my grandmother to the hospital and five days later on Christmas morning she passed away. I blamed myself for it. What if I checked on her like I should have? What if I paid more attention to her? All these questions plagued my mind and it took a toll on me. Even though the doctors said that no matter the time she got to the hospital she had a low chance of surviving, I put that blame on myself.

It was time for me to go back to school and start the outdoor track season. I was excited yet sad at the same time. I just lost my grandmother but I had to stay strong so I could get back into the competitive mindset. The semester started out fine until one night, a month after my grandmother's passing, I received an email saying that a good friend of mine from home was found shot and killed in the back seat of his car. Again, being young I didn't know how to process all of this and I never spoke about my feelings to anyone. I did what I did best and kept it bottled up inside and tried to brush it off.

With all these events occurring, it started to affect my practices and my actions. I wasn't thinking straight. This isn't supposed to be happening to me at such a young age. When the time came for my first track meet, I didn't even want to run. For the first time, I felt defeated before I stepped on the track. After the track meet I made the decision to transfer back home and run on my own. I was going to transfer to the University of South Carolina – Upstate and become an independent runner. So, I put in my application, got accepted, and moved back home.

The one thing that kept me happy was knowing I had a loving girlfriend waiting for me to come home. I was excited to be back with her and see what would happen. However, soon after coming home that summer, she called me and ended things. I was supposed to pick her up that afternoon after church, but she told me she couldn't be with me anymore. I was completely heartbroken, and it pushed me over the edge. I just lost three people I loved and cared for in a six-month period. I still wouldn't talk about it, so everything continued to eat me up inside.

My world was crashing down on me. The more I thought about everything that happened, the more I dug myself into a hole. It was hard to believe that all of this was true, and the only way I felt I could cope was to stop caring. I started to lose trust in myself and in others. I didn't want to be close to anyone, so I started to slowly shut everyone out.

NOTES

Hitting Rock Bottom

*Nothing is given to man on earth, struggle is
built into the nature of life.*

~Andrew Bernstein

Going from being so relentless and feeling like
nothing can stop me to hitting rock bottom was not
something I had planned for my life. Does anyone
ever plan for that? I was so unprepared for this down-
ward spiral in my life and it changed me for the
worse. I still planned on running independently and
competing on my own, but the fire was not there anymore, the motivation to keep going was not there
anymore. Then one day I woke up to a torn patellar
tendon in my knee. For me that was my last hope of
doing anything great with my life.

The injury took me out for a few weeks and once
I was able to get back on the track, I had no will or
desire to. I told myself well maybe I can just focus
on school and go from there. What many people
don't know about me is that I am a musician. I started
playing piano when I was about eleven and just became good at it. I never learned to read sheet music;

I learned everything by ear. One of my ideas was that if I was never able to make it as a runner, maybe I could make it as a musician. I picked piano back up hoping it would give me a little satisfaction in my life.

The more the days went by the more depressed I became. Everything I was hiding was continuing to eat at me, but I still refused to talk about it. I never exposed my guilt concerning my grandmother. It got to the point where I didn't care about school. I was skipping class, not studying, and it showed in my grades. I finally got put on academic probation where if I didn't have a certain grade average by the end of the semester, I would lose my financial aid.

My parents stayed worried about me. This is not the son they raised to be successful, this is not the son they raised to never give up, to never quit. The sad truth was that I was slipping slowly. I constantly argued with my parents because I didn't want to be in the wrong. What I was doing was perfectly fine; no one could tell me what to do. I started losing friends because of this. I was in so much pain that I took it out on everyone who got close to me. I would get into a relationship, but once I felt like it was growing, I would end it. I didn't want to be in the position to lose anyone else.

Finally, I gave up on school and decided to pursue a career in music. I took a semester off from school to try to make it in music and my parents told me if I wanted to do that, they were going to start charging rent for me to live with them. I was this big bad guy that knew what he was doing and had it all figured out, so I told them I would do it. At the time I was working a part-time job, but because I took a semester off school I had to work full-time to pay my parents. I took on more hours and began my "music career."

The pain continued to grow inside of me, I didn't know who I was becoming and it scared me. I felt alone, I felt scared, I felt beat up. Even though my parents were there and trying to help me, I refused it. I was out to prove a point which came back to slap me in the face. I did a couple of music gigs here and there, but I did not put in enough effort to even get recognized. I thought it was going to be easy and everyone would be calling to have me perform. Everyone tried to tell me that it was hard, but I didn't want to hear that.

The number of bad days continued to grow. I started getting careless with my money. Being responsible became less and less of a habit. I would get bank statements saying I was in overdraft, but it wasn't my fault, it was the bank's fault. This led to many arguments with my parents and the more we argued the angrier I became; the only problem is I didn't know what I was angry at. I just had to be right. I would go the gym to work out, but once I got there I would do a couple exercises, lose interest, then leave. Nobody knew my pain because I refused to let anybody in. I was literally at rock bottom.

NOTES

The End is Near

I'm told to stay strong, keep fighting; but they don't understand...I've already lost.

~Unknown

Hitting rock bottom is like hitting a dead end to your life. It's a feeling of nothingness and emptiness. You start having thoughts that things would be better off if you weren't around. That is the exact thought I had on a particular day. The night before I had an argument with my dad, but I don't remember what it was about. We argued so much that it all became a big blur.

I woke up like I usually do, had breakfast and headed off to work. On my way to work I finally broke down. All the pain, all the suffering, and all the anger caught up to me. I thought to myself this is it, I am done with life. I am getting nowhere and all I am doing is causing pain to everyone around me. At that moment I believed that if I took my life then it would be best; life would be better if I wasn't in it. I was going to kill myself, I was going to drive my car off a bridge or off the road. I was so selfish that I didn't even care about others' well-being.

I started to call everyone to apologize before I took that leap. In the back of my mind, I was hoping someone cared enough to stop me but also, I wanted to apologize for all the pain I caused. Right as I was ready to take my life my friend Samer Hosn called. Sam and I had been great friends for years since high school. He called me back after missing my call and I was in tears. I was spilling everything out to him. He tried everything he could to calm me down and he eventually got me to pull over. Once I got off the phone with Sam, I called my mom and she told me to stay put so she could come get me.

I was so angry with myself I couldn't take my grip off the steering wheel. I squeezed that steering wheel like my life depended on it. I cried and cried and screamed in pain. All the years of suffering and years of holding my guilt in, plus the loss of loved ones came out and it felt like a burden was lifted off my chest. I was no longer suffocating; I was no longer screaming on the inside. I had given a voice to my pain.

NOTES

Redeemed

I do not seek redemption from the conse-quences of my sin. I seek to be redeemed from sin itself. Until I have attained that end, I shall be content to be restless.

~Mahatma Gandhi

What does it mean to be redeemed? According to Merriam-Webster Dictionary, redeemed means "to extricate from or help to overcome something detrimental" or to "atone or make amends for." Either way, it leads to the same path of recovery, making changes that will be for the better, steering away from any negativity. To be redeemed of something is to be cleansed of any wrong or sinful nature.

Personally, to be redeemed is to have a fresh start. When I decided I wanted to get better, I wanted to redeem myself by becoming a better man. I wanted to put the path I was headed if I didn't get help, be-hind me. Many times, you will hear me say, "When your legacy is on the line, you fight for it." I feel that to be true in any situation. I was at the point to where

I was fighting for my life because I had entered a dark place where I had become blind.

Becoming redeemed is not something that happens overnight, but over time. It is countless hours in a day you spend taking care of yourself. This will come with many challenges, many tests. Sometimes, the only way we can succeed and move forward is by having setbacks and failures. It's up to you to decide how you want to proceed. Slow, steady progress is better than no progress. Having the strength to stand up when you get knocked down.

Being redeemed is to be bound by purpose. What do I mean by that? What does it mean to be bound by purpose? It means there is a reason you were put on this earth. There are two times in your life you know have a purpose, the day you were born and the day you figure out why. We all have a purpose in life whether we believe it or not. Your purpose is what allows you to continue forward in your journey. To be redeemed is to have purpose. I had no clue what my purpose was in life. I had no clue where I was headed. But I knew I was bound by purpose.

Redemption can come in the form of a second chance. Only we can control our destiny, but we all have a chance to re-create our reason behind the change. Each person who looks to be redeemed has the opportunity to rewrite their story. The opportunity to be someone other than what we were once perceived to be. We often lose sight of who we really are. The light becomes dim in our minds as well as our imaginations. Our only hope is redemption. Being able to wake up every day and say, "Hey! This is me!" and be proud of it.

My final thought on becoming redeemed doesn't necessarily come in the form of religion or a belief system. One often thinks that in order to become redeemed, you must accept some sort of a higher power. Being a Christian myself, I do not believe that statement to be true. I believe in order to become redeemed; you must believe in yourself. Rid the toxins from within that eat away at your soul and fight the biggest fight of your life. Only you control your destiny. No one else but you! Having a faith system is helpful in keeping on track. I definitely used one and will forever use one.

NOTES

Recovery is a Process

The real challenge of growth, mentally, emotionally, and spiritually comes when you get knocked down. It takes courage to act. Part of being hungry when you've been defeated. It takes courage to start over again.

~Les Brown

That night my mom, dad, and I sat down, and I poured everything out. They started to realize the problem was not with them, it wasn't with my friends, and it was all with me. I finally admitted to the guilt of blaming myself for my grandmother's death. Also, the loss of my best friend and girlfriend played a role in my pain. My mom gave me two options: I could either seek help from church or she was going to put me in a program. I chose to seek help from church. I started to see the associate pastor, David Smith, every Friday for an hour.

My associate pastor and I had a lot in common so it was easier to open up to him and talk things out. Every session we would pray, he would ask me what was on my mind, then we would basically just talk sports and working out. He became such a tremendous help and impact to getting me back on the right track, but I had a ways to go. I still needed a plan that would guide me to the right direction and get me back on my feet. I still had my days of doubt, but the more help I got the easier it became.

Recovery is not something that comes overnight, just like anything else it takes work and dedication. The way I saw it, either I can treat it as a challenge or I can see it as a process. So I put them together. I wanted to challenge myself to not only get better but to improve each week. I had to trust the process. Of course, there were still bumps and setbacks along the way, but instead of giving up I kept pushing forward. Things slowly started to progress with my parents and my friends, but the one thing I still struggled with was relationships. I still had that fear of loss of a loved one.

The very next semester I started back in school and was put back on academic probation. But I had something to prove to myself. I took each day as its own, not trying to look at the long-term goals but more of the short term. I found by doing that, my recovery was better. It helped build my confidence. I still felt depressed some days but by also getting back in the gym, I was able to tackle it and move forward. It was amazing how much energy I had and how much better I felt after starting the recovery process.

Some days I would get a little aggravated knowing I had a long road ahead of me. I was so far behind in school and wasn't sure what my plan was, so I would just get upset. Each day was a new challenge. I started making better grades and was actually enjoying school. I was getting some of that mental toughness back that I had when I was in high school and before the events started to happen. I continued to see my associate pastor on Fridays for about a year until we felt like I was strong enough. He always told me his door was open if I needed him which made me feel good knowing I had the option.

My relationship with my parents was improving. Me and my dad still bickered about different things, but it was more of which of us can be more stubborn over a project or him trying to educate me about something. I was young, still made mistakes along the way but I was learning from them and taking advice. One thing my mom has always told me is that I get my stubbornness from my dad. I get my strengths from my dad. The more I think about it the more I understand as to why he would push me so hard to be great. He wanted to see me succeed. My mom did as well, and she had no issue with threatening to beat my butt if needed.

All things considered I was headed in the right direction to becoming better and getting my head on straight. I was finally taken off academic probation, but I had already lost any scholarships I had in place. I was feeling more alive with more work to do. The only real thing that kept me from feeling complete was my ability to compete on the track. I lost all motivation when that happened and to this day I kick myself for it.

NOTES

God Loves You

Have I not commanded you? Be strong and courageous. Do not be afraid; do not be discouraged, for the LORD your God will be with you wherever you go.

~Joshua 1:9 (NIV)

One thing that I have never been afraid to admit, is that I am a Christian. I believe in the Lord and even when I was going through my worst times, I still looked to him for help. Soon after I started my recovery process, I was severely tested. The same year I started the healing process, my mom was diagnosed with breast cancer. The first thing that came to mind was here we go again. Is this never going to end? But because I was trying to remain strong, that is exactly what I did. I told myself, this is a true test of how strong I can become.

I remember being at work one day talking to a customer. We had just got done working on his car and I was handing him his paperwork when he looked at me, shook my hand and said, "God loves you." At first, I just kind of brushed it off and didn't think much of it. I get told that all the time, so this didn't seem any different. On my way home that night it hit me what that gentleman told me. For some reason when I replayed that conversation in my head and let it sink in what he said, I felt an instant release of stress like no other. I had never felt this way before and it let me know everything was going to be ok with my mom. I knew at that point everything was going to be ok.

My mom was diagnosed October 2008 and had surgery that December, which was around the time we had finals and exams at school. Trying to juggle studying with being concerned about my mom was challenging. I didn't know how I was going to do it. What I did know is that I was going to stay strong for my mom and finish my semester strong. After my mom had her surgery she immediately started radiation treatment. She went for six straight weeks and it took a toll on her body, but she is such a tough woman. She battled and conquered cancer and to this day she is cancer-free. Seeing my mom be tough gave me hope that I can overcome any obstacle that came my way because I was her son and she raised me that way.

With the mixture of stress and depression I was overcoming a new nightmare that came with it called anxiety. It slowly started creeping in, starting with waking up nervous. I began to lose sleep due to the fear of waking up nervous and being sick to my stomach. I wasn't eating due to the anxiety, which caused me to lose weight. There were a couple of times I had to be taken to the hospital because I would hyperventilate. This went on a couple of weeks before I decided to see my doctor. At that point I was diagnosed with anxiety and depression.

My doctor prescribed Xanax and Zoloft to help ease the tension. I took it as prescribed and it helped for a little bit, but eventually the anxiety became too strong for me to handle and the medicine only worked for a portion of the time. My anxiety had progressed and turned into sleep paralysis which meant I had anxiety attacks in my sleep. It felt like I was being suffocated in my dreams, but my body wouldn't wake up. When I eventually woke up, I didn't know where I was and I was sweating from being out of breath.

The level of anxiety took such a toll on me it created issues in every area of my life. I began to have anxiety attacks during work and my body would cramp up. I couldn't move, I could barely breathe, it was like fighting for air. One time I had an anxiety attack while driving. It started in my hands and moved through my body. The muscles in my hands contracted and I couldn't open my hands back up. It was a total nightmare. Not being in control when I had anxiety attacks was affecting my entire life.

The only thing that kept me going was remembering what the stranger told me that day, "God loves you." My limits were severely tested and I prevailed because I knew I had to stay strong, not only for myself but for my parents. Even though I was suffering, I had to continue to push forward. My only issue was how am I going tackle anxiety without it bringing me down? I found myself constantly being tested in and outside of school while anxiety took shots at me. I battled with being able to maintain a stable relationship. I was getting everything thrown my way. How would I be able to tackle it all?

NOTES

Embarking a New Journey

You can't connect the dots looking forward; you can only connect them looking backwards. So you have to trust that the dots will somehow connect in your future. You have to trust in something – your gut, destiny, life, karma, whatever. Because believing that the dots will connect down the road will give you the confidence to follow your heart even when it leads you off the well-worn path; and that will make all the difference.

~Steve Jobs

One of the biggest questions I would ask myself is what can I do to get my competitive edge back? At this point in my life I had gotten big into working out and lifting weights. My last couple years of college I became a fitness freak. If I wasn't in the classroom, I was in the gym. It was a great way for me to release stress and to get back into phenomenal shape. I knew I wanted to do something with health and fitness as a career, so I studied exercise science as my major. I loved the anatomy of the human body. Anything related to science and biology fascinated me and I excelled at it.

After graduating with a four-year degree, I was working two jobs. I was a physical therapist aide and a personal trainer. I enjoyed doing both but eventually the aide job turned into an as-needed basis so my focus was the gym. I loved being able to help others become better and feel better. Working in the gym was also where I realized I had a way of getting my competitive edge back. I got into Olympic lifting and power lifting and challenged myself to get stronger. It got to the point where I was challenging my friends to a lift off and car pulling. It made me feel alive and provided a challenge which was something I was missing out on in my life.

I got so involved in the gym my friend Sam asked me why I didn't compete. It was something I had thought about but wasn't sure if I was ready to take it to that level. About this time was when I met my wife, Megan Elmore. She joined the gym around the same time I started to work there. At the time I wasn't looking for a relationship because I was still building myself up and I also had the fear of heartbreak. When I tried dating before, I kept getting my heart broke, so I gave up on it. Megan would come in and what started out as a couple months of teasing and just friendly talk, turned into more.

I remember she would come in and I would always tell her she was late and needed to get it together. I was still working for the physical therapy company when we met so I invited her to our Christmas dinner party. I still wasn't sure what I wanted at the time. I had become a closed book when it came to relationships, but somehow, she kept tearing down this wall I had up and found her way in. We spent more and more time together, and I started to think maybe she's the one although I still had a big fear of losing another person in my life. I took it day by day. I definitely made mistakes within the relationship but I had to learn and grow from it.

When I decided I wanted to compete I had no clue where I needed to start. I didn't know what to expect but just like track it was something I learned along the way. Megan was always excited about what I was doing in the gym. Her father, Joe Elmore, had a trainer, BJ Little that he met with once a week. Megan was telling me all about BJ and how I needed to meet him. When I finally met BJ we immediately hit it off. We both shared the same passion of fitness and he also was a college athlete. BJ was an all-American linebacker and had the utmost knowledge in strength training.

I told BJ my idea of competing in a power lift competition and asked his advice on how to build my strength. He gave me advice but one time I asked him if we could have a training session and that's all it took. From that point on we met once a week to train and we had about eight months to get ready for my first competition. What started off as BJ training me turned into a friendship. He was able to bring the relentlessness back that I was looking for. He took me at my worst and made me my best and I am forever thankful for that.

NOTES

The Start of a Comeback

If you take responsibility for yourself you will develop a hunger to accomplish your dreams.

~Les Brown

Preparing for my first competition was very stressful. Finding the time to train and wondering if I was good enough to compete would really weigh me down. But BJ would be there to guide me in the right direction which is what I needed. We trained hard for eight months and each week I felt myself improving and getting stronger. It was good education too for me because it gave me more insight on how I could improve my workouts when BJ wasn't around.

The day had finally come. The day I had been training and working hard for - competition day. I still wasn't sure what to expect since it was my first competition, but I knew that I was there to win. I was competing in three different events: power curl, bench press, and dead lifts. Like any lifter, you start looking around at other lifters to see who your biggest competition might be, but not everyone was in the same weight class and division. The WNPF (World National Powerlift Federation) had different classes you could be a part of. For me, I was in the novice 181 weight class.

My mind was racing, and my nerves were high, just like it was when I ran track. This was a way for me to make my comeback in the competitive world and I was determined to be the best. I went out and I gave it my all; I hit all three lift attempts in each event and came out on top in each event in my division and weight class. At that moment I knew I had found a way to redeem myself. I talked to BJ and told him I wanted to continue to compete and be a world champion. From that point we had started a brotherhood that no one could break.

I remember being in shock when they gave me the best lifter award. For my first competition to win overall in my division and come home with the best lifter award, I didn't know what to think. I had dedicated this competition to my mom for her battle with breast cancer. I wanted to win for her to show my strength to overcome and get back to becoming a champion. To me this was a comeback of a lifetime.

The next competition I trained for was a little more challenging because it was the national qualifier. I had a chance to compete for the national power lift title. Just to say I qualified was a big deal for me.

BJ and I started training and he really started to step up the difficulty of training. I always came home feeling beat up, which is part of being a power lifter; being able to push your body to the absolute limits. I got asked all the time: "Why do you put your body through that?" "Why do you continue to train if you are hurting?" Nobody understood why I was able push through the pain and injuries.

My wife would constantly worry about me, but she stood by my side all the way through it. There were times she had to help me get upstairs, help me shower, and bring the food to bed because I was in so much pain I couldn't move. It didn't matter what others thought or felt because I was doing this for me. It was my way of getting back what I lost all those years. If I wasn't going to be a world champion track star, I was going to be a world champion power lifter. I did what it took to be a champion.

There were days I didn't feel like working out because I felt depressed. I felt so down on myself, I could barely lift the weight. There were days I just didn't feel strong and I would get so mad and throw my lifting belt because what should be easy felt hard. But BJ reminded me that it is only practice. Nobody is here to see the hard work you put in, they only see the end result which is what matters most. In the weight room I had to lift the weight so many reps, but on the platform, I would only have to lift it once.

NOTES

Raising the Bar

I'm pissed off for greatness. Because if you ain't pissed off for greatness, that means you're OK with being mediocre.

~Ray Lewis

One of the things about being a power lifter, as I said in the previous chapter, is the pain you must overcome. Why put yourself through that? The more I trained the more I started asking myself that same question. Is it worth feeling this way the rest of my life? But because it was a way for me to redeem myself, I told myself, yes, it's completely worth it.

For six months BJ and I trained to get ready for the national qualifier meet. I was starting to feel like my old self again. I was determined to become better. Nothing was standing in my way this time. I had one goal in mind and that was to become the World Champion. First, I had to qualify to get there. We took each day one step at a time with my training. I was feeling stronger and unstoppable at this point. It was time to qualify for nationals and I was feeling confident.

One thing BJ would always harp on was for me to be smart when it came closer to competition days. Well it was the last week before competition and I was getting my final lift preparation in, so I decided I was going to pull my car to finish my workout. I got hooked up to the car, got my first pull in and went to reset for the next. I got all the way to the finish when the cord snapped and popped me in the back of my leg. It put me on the ground and sounded like a shotgun went off. Luckily it just did exterior damage to my leg and bottom but still added an extreme amount of pain. I was more worried about telling BJ than I was about my leg because I knew he would not be happy with me. The next week was competition week so I nursed my leg and I actually got lucky it didn't keep me from competing. Matter of fact, I never felt it at all after that day.

The national qualifier was one of the most intense days of my competitive career. I felt so much pressure to qualify but as always, I would use that towards my lifts. When your adrenaline is high you can lift more than you think you can. You underestimate your abilities some. I went in and I knew the lifts I needed to hit so I concentrated on just that. The top three in each event went to the national qualifier so if I could just get enough to qualify I could put everything I had into the National Championships.

This was such a huge deal to me even if it wasn't to others. I had to prove to myself I still had what it takes.

The moment had come to step on the platform and I was feeling confident. There is nothing like stepping onto the lifting platform and grabbing that bar before a lift. Something would come over me that is hard to explain, but for an instant I felt at ease and when the judge gave me the lift command I would rip that weight up with everything I had. I had the same feeling before every track event. I would sit in the blocks and for that one second before the gun went off I would get that feeling of easement. The only difference now is I am on a lifting platform instead of a track.

I battled all day and qualified in each event to go to the USA Power Lift meet. The feeling I had was so incredible. For the first time in a long time I felt like I was accomplishing something in my life. I was getting one step closer to the world title I was hungry for since I was little. At this point we knew I had to step it up a little more in the weight room to take the USA title, So BJ and I went back to the gym and took it up another notch.

NOTES

Pain is Temporary

Pain is temporary. It may last a minute, or an hour, or a day, or a year, but eventually it will subside and something else will take its place. If I quit, however, it lasts forever.

~Lance Armstrong

At this point in my career I was so ambitious. I was rebuilding a legacy I never was able to finish. I was making a name for myself. I had three months to train for the USA power lift championships. The only way I knew I could win was to really take it to the next level and train like I have never trained before. BJ at this point wanted me to work more on form instead of strength because my deadlift form was not the best. He said if I improved my deadlift form I would become even stronger in that event.

At this time, I asked my friend Katie Turner to start filming my workouts because I wanted to capture those moments and start making motivational videos. It was also a good way for me to go back and look at my form and see the improvements I was making. I felt so indestructible that I would tell BJ to keep bringing everything he had. I wanted to be the very best and so we trained as if I was the very best. In the back of my mind I still had that fear of losing. I hadn't lost up to this point.

The day things took a turn was the day I injured my hamstring a month out from the USA power lift competition. We were doing dead lift repeats, fairly heavy, and on the last set I got the bar an inch off the ground and my hamstring popped. I dropped, and I couldn't believe what had just happened. All it took was that one moment to end what took me months to prepare for. As I laid there BJ and Katie tried to help me get comfortable and all I could think was is this it for me?

I started to hyperventilate from being in so much pain. BJ was running around trying to find something to help and Katie was trying to calm me down. But the most dreaded part was calling my wife, Megan. Her biggest fear was getting a phone call that I had hurt myself. Amy Bogan, the gym nurse and my friend, was able to wrap my leg with ice and help BJ carry me out to Megan's car. I remember looking at BJ and asking, "I can still compete right?" I could tell BJ was upset and felt responsible. But there was nothing he could have done to prevent it. It was a freak injury and it was bound to happen eventually.

We got to the doctor's office and BJ met us there so we could figure out what happened. At this point I was able to control my breathing and relax some, but my leg was in so much pain I couldn't straighten it out. We finally spoke with the doctor and just as expected I was out of the competition. I tore my hamstring and it wouldn't heal in time for me to participate. After we left the doctor's office it sunk in that all the hard work I put in was over in one second. It was recommended that I never compete again and that is not something I was prepared to accept.

The next few weeks I felt sorry for myself and the more I thought about it the more it made me angry I couldn't compete. One thing that kept me positive was all the support I had from gym members, my friends, my wife, and BJ. Even though I wasn't competing anymore I still had hope for greatness. So many times I asked myself what if I hadn't got hurt, where would I be? Would I have won?

A couple months later I was on the WNPF website and I noticed I still had a chance to compete at the World Championships. I never wanted to end my career like I had. Of course, I asked Megan if she was ok with it and she told me she would support me in whatever I decided to do, so I called BJ and asked him if it was possible. He said let's go for it, so I started preparing for the biggest platform once again.

NOTES

Mental Strength vs. Physical Strength

Knowing is not enough, we must apply. Willing is not enough, we must do.

~Bruce Lee

Being back in the gym training for the biggest moment in my life gave me back that satisfaction I was missing for two months when I wasn't competing. I started rehabbing my leg while also trying to prepare for the World Championships. BJ and I both agreed I would just compete in the power curl event since my leg wasn't close to being ready. I only had one month to train, which really isn't enough time considering the circumstances. But, because I was hungry for this title, I did what I had to do.

We trained for the limited time that we had and made the best of it. I was feeling confident that I could reach that level of competitiveness and it was the only thing on my mind. Again, I was so thankful to have BJ there to lead me in the right direction. I wouldn't have been where I was in my career if it wasn't for him. I did what he asked so that I could improve my strength not only in my mind but in the power curl.

The day came to qualify for the World Championships and I went in like it was any other competition; confident and ready to win. I needed to get first place to qualify. The power curl was the first event, so I went in and hit all three attempts setting a new state record. I had done it. I qualified for the world championships. I couldn't wait to get started with training, but again, I only had one month to prepare, so I had to really be smart with my training.

I continued strengthening my leg while still preparing for the world championships. Even though I wasn't dead lifting, I could still feel the pain in my leg while performing the power curl. Recovery was very tough but if I wanted to win I had to suck it up and push through the pain to overcome one of the biggest obstacles I've ever faced. Training was tough because I felt worn out from the previous competition, so it set me back a little. I wasn't sure if I was going to be ready and it showed come competition day.

The day came for the World Power Lift Competition in Atlanta, Georgia. I was excited but extremely nervous at the same time. It was a different level of competing, but I believed if I could pull it off, I would redeem myself from my past. When I say I was nervous, that is an understatement. Looking at what I was up against, the top lifters of the world, I started to get in my head too much. I had myself defeated before the meet started. Since I was only doing Power Curl, I wouldn't get the results until the very end of the day. The only thing I knew was I had to win.

The meet started, and I was sweating. My brother, Josh Stephens, was with me trying to get me calm and keep me pumped at the same time. The more and more I thought about it, the more I started to doubt myself and overthink my lifts. Am I starting at the right weight? What If I don't get my attempts? My mind was racing a hundred miles an hour. My first attempt was a good lift, but something didn't feel right; I didn't feel as strong. I went for my second attempt and failed. At this point I had already lost and as I did my last attempt, I failed again.

I blew the biggest competition and I felt like such a failure. I allowed the pressure of winning and breaking the world power curl record to take away my ability to be my best. My dad came up to me and hugged me because he knew I was upset. My parents always supported me when I allowed them to. As much as they worried about me, they still came. After the meet was over I went back to my hotel room and replayed everything in my head. It wasn't the last of me, I was determined to get that title. I got up, went back to the drawing board and pushed forward.

NOTES

Fighting for my Legacy

We get one opportunity in life, one chance at life to do whatever you're going to do and lay your foundation and make whatever mark you're going to make. Whatever legacy you're going to leave; leave your legacy!

~Ray Lewis

Something I always tell everyone is that power lifting is not always about physical strength. There is a lot of emotion that goes into every practice and every meet. To me competing is 90% mental and 10% physical. If your mind is not in the right place, you will not be able to perform your best. That is exactly what happened to me after being defeated at World's. My mind took a plunge and I began to doubt my abilities as a lifter. I was barely able to perform lifts, my body started to wear down and it affected my workouts.

In the back of my mind I was still the best and wanted to prove to myself that I could become the World's Best. Even though I had doubt, I still gave it my all. One thing I have always told myself is if I don't feel like 100%, I will at least give 100% of how I feel that day. I had two competitions lined up before heading back to the World Championships for a redemption round, but this time I was going to have a different mindset. My legacy was on the line and I was going to fight for it.

The first competition came up, and again since my leg wasn't 100% I only continued to do the power curl. I started to feel myself getting burned out with the power curl because it was all I was doing. It started to take a toll on my motivation to compete as well. I won the first competition but only hit two attempts out of three. I was trying to figure a way out of my slump. It felt like something was missing, like I needed something to spark to get me back on my feet and get my fire back.

I continued to train, but one thing was more important than anything else - this was the year I got married. On May 25th, 2015, Megan and I got married and there was no better feeling than this. She had stuck it out with me at my worse and best times and I was happy to have her by my side. This was the best day of my life. Nothing else could take that away either. We got married and had an amazing honeymoon although I was sick the entire time. Even through all the pain and suffering I had in the past years, she was able to make it all better and for that I was ready to spend the rest of my life with her.

After coming back from the honeymoon, I had to get back into training mode. BJ and I continued to train hard and try to figure out ways to get me back on track with the fire I needed. I was starting to doubt myself again and come down on myself hard. My leg was still hurting, and I knew if I didn't find a way to step it up I was going to fail. BJ had to constantly remind me that I was just practicing which was the hardest part. The hard work will show when I step on the platform.

The USA championships was my next challenge and competition. I knew since I missed it the previous year because of my injury that I had to do well here. As I was going through weigh-ins and giving Troy, the WNPF owner, my weight attempts I asked him what I needed to do to deadlift at World's. He told me I would need to qualify at this competition. I hadn't deadlifted in a year and wasn't sure if my leg was ready, but I had no choice but to deadlift if I wanted a chance at the world title other than power curl.

Competition day came, and I was feeling a little more confident then I had in the past competition but still had it in my mind that I could fail. The meet started and I hit my first two attempts in power curl but failed my final attempt. My biggest fear and obstacle came when it was time to deadlift. Again, I didn't know what to expect of my leg and if it was ready, but I had to at least do enough to qualify. I went to do my first attempt and it felt difficult, but I was able to succeed. I tested my leg and added more weight to the next attempt. I had success, so I added more weight in the final attempt. I never felt so much power than I did after that last attempt. I was successful at my final attempt and I immediately felt the fire come back. It was what I needed to get back in the game and become confident again. Now I was ready to take on the World Championships!

NOTES

Becoming the
World Champion

*I hated every minute of training, but I said,
'Don't quit. Suffer now and live the rest of
your life as a champion.'*

~Muhammad Ali

After competing and taking the win in the USA
Power Lift Competition, I had more confidence going into the World Championships than the previous
year. Being able to deadlift without any leg pain gave
me a boost of confidence because it brought that fire
back that was missing. I trained hard and rehabili-
tated my leg to withstand the amount of weight I
would need to lift to win the championships. This
was my year to redeem myself and take the World
Championship Title.

I trained hard and smart so that I didn't reinjure
my leg. The thought still ran through the back of my
mind and I was nervous that I would reinjure while
preparing. But I had a goal and mission and I wasn't
going to back down until I knew I had it. I had more

time to train this round so BJ and I came up with a system that would allow me to push myself hard but also allow me to back off in order to let my leg rest. We trained twice as hard and with a more focused mind I could tell a difference in how my workouts had improved and my mindset was more positive.

The day had come for me to compete for the World Title. We went down on a Friday for weigh-ins and after I made weight I went and carb-loaded, like I always do, and then spent the rest of the night getting my mindset right. The only concern I had was that my lower back and leg were causing some pain and discomfort but nothing I couldn't handle. When I woke up the next morning I immediately put my headphones on and got in my pre-competition zone.

When I compete I get dead quiet, I don't speak to anyone. I came to finish what I started. I had a different feeling than the previous year. I wasn't in my head, I felt a positive wave throughout my body. I was loose, I was confident, and shockingly wasn't nervous. My adrenaline was pumping but I was ready to step on that platform and show the world that I was the best. I feared no one that day. BJ kept me motivated and kept me on the edge which is exactly what I needed. He got me that far and it was time for us to finish strong.

The power curl was the first event and I was feeling strong. I came up for the first attempt and easily lifted it for a good lift. I actually felt like I could have the world record. My second attempt came and once again easily lifted it up for a good lift. Only one lift stood in my way from being able to attempt the world record. The world record at the time was 185 pounds, so I would have needed to curl 190 pounds to take the world record in the weight class. The bar was loaded, and I went to attempt my third lift, unfortunately, my final attempt was red-lighted for improper form and I did not get to attempt for the world record. I was ok with that because I came out to win and I felt like my first two attempts were enough for that.

I had time before I had to deadlift, so I made sure that I stayed loose and remained focused. I still had a little concern about my leg and lower back pain that was pulsing but at this point it didn't matter, I was going after the title. We stretched, and I kept food in my system to make sure my energy level didn't drop. For anyone who has never competed, if you let your adrenaline lower, it's almost impossible to get it back. Adrenaline is what helps gives you an extra boost and you always end up lifting more than you expected.

It was time for me deadlift and I was ready. I was warmed up, loose, and ready to be unleashed. It was time for my first attempt. When I stepped up and grabbed the bar, I could tell at that moment I was going to be able to lift it. My first attempt was a success. Second attempt came and at this point my nerves were starting to run high. The second attempt determined how much my leg could handle for the final attempt. I grabbed the bar and stood straight up with it no problem and had a good lift. When it came down to the final attempt, I was feeling good and knew I could lock this title in. They loaded the bar as I kneeled, imagining myself lift the weight. The bar was loaded and this was it. I walked up to the bar as I told myself, "I got this, I got this." I grabbed the bar, took a deep breath, lifted the bar and set it down. I look up and saw the three white lights and that moment I knew what I had just did. I screamed in excitement.

It was at that very moment that I became the World Champion. I remember going to the bathroom to wash the chalk off my hands and when I came out BJ was there, and we said to each other, "We did it!" I just overcame the biggest setback of my life to become the World Champion. Through all the depression, anxiety, and attempted suicide, I was able to bounce back and re-claim my legacy. No one knows this, not even my wife until now, I went back

to the hotel room and I cried at what I had just ac-
complished. To come from rock bottom and thoughts
of taking my own life to become the best in the world
- my legacy was now complete.

NOTES

Reflection

*Let me tell you something you already know.
The world ain't all sunshine and rainbows. It
is a very mean and nasty place and it will beat
you to your knees and keep you there perma-
nently if you let it. You, me, or nobody is
gonna hit as hard as life. But it ain't how hard
you hit; it's about how hard you can get hit,
and keep moving forward. How much you can
take and keep moving forward. That's how
winning is done.*

~Rocky Balboa

One of the biggest things I could ever take away from my past is to never give up, no matter how tough things get. I see too many individuals out there quitting at the first signs of a struggle. They make it a habit and it becomes a lifestyle. One of the biggest advice I can give someone who is going through the struggles of anxiety and depression, is to get up and fight! Remember who you are and where you came from. There is nothing more powerful than the power of one's own mind. You can't and must refuse to give up at any obstacle. Find a way to hurdle it! Embrace the nature of your being! It all starts with a vision and a mindset, but you must become obsessed with that vision. No one is ever going make something happen for you, you must go out and get it for yourself.

Being an example of what it is like to make the biggest comeback of one's life, it brings me a sense of power knowing I can overcome anything. As I said in previous chapters, you may not feel 100%, but you will give 100% of how you feel that day. We are going to have days we feel like giving up, feel like throwing in the towel, but you must not give in to the temptation of such negative behavior. How will you ever succeed if you have never taken a step forward? Staying in your comfort zone will only get you so far! Feeling sorry for yourself will only get you so far! We are the writers, creators, and directors of our own story. How do you want to be remembered? How do you want your reputation to stand before you?

Becoming a champion is about the willingness to Grind to Conquer. Make peace with the pain. Be accountable. Understanding you will either be the biggest part of your own success, or the biggest obstacle in the way. Never take for granted the tools set before you to succeed and never let anyone stand in your way. Never let anyone tell you what you are not capable of. Show them exactly what you are capable of! Never let anyone tell you that you are overly passionate about anything. If you're passionate about something, never be sorry. Keep pushing toward your dreams and let others dwell in your success. Stay forever hungry!

NOTES

Depression & Anxiety Statistics

Based on surveys and findings of the ADAA (Anxiety and Depression Association of America)

As many might know, depression and anxiety can run together. This means if someone is suffering from depression, they are more likely to suffer from anxiety as well or vice versa. Depression and anxiety are the biggest mental illnesses in the U.S. today and many people go untreated. Most causes are from a chemical imbalance. Without proper treatment, it could lead to higher stress, lower motivation and/or suicidal thoughts.

According to the ADAA (Anxiety and Depression Association of America) anxiety and depression affects up to 40 million adults in the U.S. age 18 or older. Only 36.9% receive treatment. Also, according to the ADAA, those suffering from anxiety and depression are three to five times more likely to visit the doctor and six times more likely to be hospital-ized than those who don't suffer from anxiety and depression.

A few disorders that can lead to high anxiety and depression are: Panic Disorders, Social Anxiety Dis-orders, Obsessive-Compulsive Disorder, and one of the biggest leading disorders; Post-traumatic Stress Disorder. Each of these are common causes that lead to anxiety and depression. Some may not realize they have these certain disorders if the signs aren't caught early or if proper treatment isn't taken.

Panic disorders can bring on heavy breathing, shaking, and loss of awareness. Based on the find-ings of ADAA, panic disorders are twice as likely to affect women than men. It affects 6 million adults or 2.7% of the U.S. population. Panic attacks can be brought on by high stress, in your sleep (night ter-rors), over thinking, and high intense situations. Panic disorders may also bring on hyperventilation, or in other words, out of control breathing.

Social Anxiety Disorders can be brought on by being in awkward situations, such as being in a crowd. Being around a lot of people you don't know can bring on high stress. It's a feeling of being judged or you don't want people looking at you. The ADAA conducted a survey back in 2007 which stated that 36% of people with SAD will experience symptoms for ten plus years before actually seeking help. It can affect 15 million adults and will typically begin around the age of 13. That's 6.8% of the U.S. population.

Obsessive-Compulsive Disorder, also known as OCD, affects 2.2 million adults (1.0% of U.S. Population) according to the ADAA findings. Symptoms can start around the age of 19 or as early as 14 years of age. It's one of the leading causes of stress and anxiety disorders. OCD can be defined as having the tendency to have excessive orderliness, perfectionism, and having great attention to detail. If something is out of order, it can cause high stress for those suffering from OCD disorder.

Lastly, Post-traumatic Stress Disorder (PTSD) is brought on by traumatic events at early ages. Sexual assaults and military at war are one of the biggest events that bring on PTSD. According to the ADAA it affects 7.7 million adults (3.5% of U.S. adults) and is more likely to affect women than men. PTSD is one of the biggest causes of depression. Some feel they are in a dark place and can't get out and can lead to suicidal thoughts.

All of these different disorders can lead to anxiety and depression if not treated properly. Depression is the leading cause of disability worldwide and almost 75% of people will go untreated causing them to take their lives. There are 1 million people who obtain this mental disorder. 1 in 13 people suffer from anxiety worldwide and it is the most common disorder brought on by certain phobias. Different treatments can include: therapy, medication, transcranial magnetic stimulation, and complementary and alternative treatment. To learn more about these statistics and findings, you can visit the ADAA website.

(https://adaa.org/about-adaa/press-room/facts-statistics)

NOTES.

ABOUT THE AUTHOR

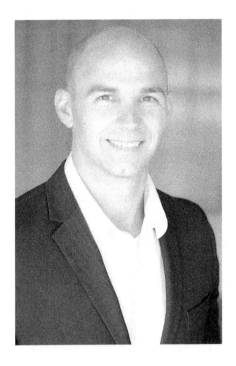

Born January 3, 1987 in Spartanburg, S.C., Daniel is the son of Alan and Cyndi Stephens, the husband of Megan Stephens and the father of Isabella Stephens. He grew up getting involved in sports and martial arts which allowed him to become very athletic and he earned his 2nd degree black belt at a young age.

Once Daniel became of age he got into track and field where he succeeded at being one of the top sprinters in the state, landing him a track scholarship at a collegiate level. He kept up with his martial arts and combat training during his off time and developed his skills more and more. Daniel also enjoys playing the piano in his free time as well and was part of a band for a short time before he decided to pursue his degree at the University of South Carolina in Exercise Science.

While obtaining his undergraduate degree, Daniel got involved in the gym during his collegiate years working hard to develop his strength and physique. He eventually landed on the Team USA WNPF Team. With two gold Medals, a national championship, several state wins, and several records under his belt, he finally retired competitive weightlifting but remained very active in the gym and body building. After making a couple of appearances on local TV shows, Daniel decided to make his way to the big screen. In February of 2018 he auditioned and was signed by Stisa Talent Agency in Spartanburg, SC. Daniel since then has worked on many projects, one being a popular TV Show, "ATL Homicide." He continues to grow and enhance his skills to become a more successful actor.

CPSIA information can be obtained
at www.ICGtesting.com
Printed in the USA
BVHW061718071019
560429BV00029B/1594/P

9 781732 870932